AQA PSYCHOLOGY A-LEVEL AND AS A STAR EXAM PAPERS.

Full mark answers to 7 past papers.

By Joseph Anthony Campbell

Copyright © 2019 by Joseph Anthony Campbell. All Rights Reserved.

All rights reserved. No part of this book may be reproduced in any form or by any electronic or mechanical means including information storage and retrieval systems, without permission in writing from the author.

Joseph Anthony Campbell.
Contact me at josephrtk@gmail.com

First Printing: November 2019.

AQA PSYCHOLOGY A-LEVEL AND AS A STAR EXAM PAPERS.

AUTHOR'S NOTE.

This book will provide you with crystal clear and accurate examples of 'A' star grade AQA AS and A level Psychology paper examinations from the new syllabus from 2016 and enables students to achieve the same grade in their upcoming examinations.

I teach both GCSE and A level Psychology and I am a qualified and experienced Psychology teacher and tutor of over 16 years standing. I teach, write and provide independent tuition in central and West London.

The resources in this book WILL help you get an A or A star in your AQA AS and A level Psychology examinations, as they have done and will continue to do so for my students.

Best wishes,

Joseph

AQA PSYCHOLOGY A-LEVEL AND AS A STAR EXAM PAPERS.

CONTENTS

Author's note. 1
CONTENTS 1
About the Author. 1
AQA AS PSYCHOLOGY (7181/1) 3
Paper 1..3
Introductory Topics in Psychology. 3
SPECIMEN MATERIAL..3
AQA AS PSYCHOLOGY (7181/1) 11
Paper 1..11
Introductory Topics in Psychology. 11
SPECIMEN MATERIAL SECOND SET..11
AQA AS PSYCHOLOGY (7181/2) 19
Paper 2 19
Psychology in Context 19
SPECIMEN MATERIAL (First set)...19
AQA AS PSYCHOLOGY (7181/2) 28
Paper 2 28
Psychology in Context 28
SPECIMEN MATERIAL (Second set) 28
AQA A-level PSYCHOLOGY (7182/1) 38
Paper 1..38
Introductory Topics in Psychology. 38
SPECIMEN MATERIAL..38
2017 38
http://filestore.aqa.org.uk/resources/psychology/AQA-71821-SQP.PDF 38
AQA A-level PSYCHOLOGY (7182/2) 51
Paper 2 51
Psychology in Context 51
SPECIMEN MATERIAL..51
2017 51
http://filestore.aqa.org.uk/resources/psychology/AQA-71822-SQP.PDF 51
AQA A-level PSYCHOLOGY (7182/3) 63
Paper 3 63
Issues and Options in Psychology...63
2017 63
Paper 3 (A-level): Specimen question paper (193.6 KB) 63
AQA A-level PSYCHOLOGY (7182/3) 65

By Joseph Anthony Campbell

Paper 3 65
Issues and Options in Psychology 65
2017 65
Paper 3 (A-level): Specimen question paper (second set) (72.7 KB) 65
AQA A-level PSYCHOLOGY (7182/3) 68
Paper 3 68
Issues and Options in Psychology 68
2017 68
Paper 3 (A-level): Specimen question paper (193.6 KB) 68
AQA A-level PSYCHOLOGY (7182/3) 70
Paper 3 70
Issues and Options in Psychology 70
2017 70
Paper 3 (A-level): Specimen question paper (second set) (72.7 KB) 70
AQA A-level PSYCHOLOGY (7182/3) 73
Paper 3 73
Issues and Options in Psychology 73
2017 73
Paper 3 (A-level): Specimen question paper (193.6 KB) 73
AQA A-level PSYCHOLOGY (7182/3) 76
Paper 3 76
Issues and Options in Psychology 76
2017 76
Paper 3 (A-level): Specimen question paper (second set) (72.7 KB) 76

ABOUT THE AUTHOR.

I graduated from the Universities of Liverpool and Leeds in Psychology and I obtained first class honours in my teacher training. I am a practicing Life Coach also and I have undertaken training in Psychotherapy and Therapeutic Counselling.

I have taught and provided private tuition for over 16 years up to University level in Psychology. I also write academic resources for the Times Educational Supplement.

By Joseph Anthony Campbell

AQA AS PSYCHOLOGY (7181/1)
PAPER 1
INTRODUCTORY TOPICS IN PSYCHOLOGY.
SPECIMEN MATERIAL

Section A
Social influence

0 1 Briefly outline and evaluate the authoritarian personality as an explanation of obedience to authority. [4 marks]

An authoritarian personality is a collection of traits developed from overly strict parenting. An authoritarian personality is more likely to be conformist and obey people of perceived higher status. It is difficult to establish cause and effect between overly strict parenting and later levels of obedience. It is also difficult to easily account for obedience of entire social groups/societies.

0 2 Read the item and then answer the question that follows.

The following article appeared in a newspaper:
Britain's views on homosexuality – the biggest social change of the last 30 years?
In the UK, views on homosexuality have changed significantly in recent times. Thirty years ago, almost two-thirds of the British public opposed same-sex relationships because they were 'morally wrong'. These days, homosexuality is accepted and the majority of British people support recent changes to the laws on gay marriage and adoption.
With reference to the article above, explain how social influence leads to social change. [6 marks]

Factors affecting minority influence include consistency, commitment and flexibility. Social change occurs as viewed in the article above when the minority view, e.g. gay rights campaigners, challenges the majority view and is eventually accepted as the majority. This relates to conformity through the processes of informational social influence and internalisation. As the majority becomes more aware of the minority, they strive to understand the minority view and may internalise their views. The influence of obedience is also shown which leads to a social norm being created i.e.'...the majority of British people support recent changes to the laws on gay marriage and adoption.' Social cryptomnesia may also occur where people forget that the majority that is occurring now was once the minority.

0 3 Describe and evaluate two studies of social influence. [12 marks]

Milgram's study used 40 male participants. They were assigned the role of 'teacher' and were shown a confederate being strapped to a pseudo-electric machine. The naive participants (NP's) had switches they were to press ranging from 15 volts to 450 volts. They were to shock the participants each time the confederate gave a wrong answer, increasing the voltage each time. The confederate gave the wrong answer each time.

The results showed that 100% of the participants went to 300 volts and 65% shocked the confederate with a 450-volt shock. This showed that when a legitimate authority figure (the psychologist in the white coat) orders a person to perform even a harmful action, they will often obey. However, the experiment lacks ecological validity as people are not normally asked to shock people. Also, the experiment is arguably ethically unsound as it caused the participants emotional distress and lacked informed consent.

Zimbardo's study aimed to find out how much people conformed to roles. He used male student participants (an androcentric study like Milgram's) and randomly assigned the roles of prisoner or guard. The prisoners were mock arrested, stripped and numbered. The prisoners and guards formed groups and the prisoners became submissive and obedient to the guards. The experiment was abandoned after 6 days. Zimbardo aimed to show how ordinary people conform readily to roles. However, this experiment took place in an artificial environment and therefore lacks ecological validity. Zimbardo also acted as the prison superintendent in this experiment which could lead to observer bias and a clear conflict of interests. He, too, also caused his participants emotional distress as his participants appeared unaware at times of their right to withdraw.

Section B
Memory

0 1 Read the item and then answer the questions that follow.

Participants in an experiment were shown a film of a robbery. The participants were then divided into two groups. One group was interviewed using a standard interview technique and the other group was interviewed using the cognitive interview technique. All participants were then given an 'accuracy score' (out of 20) based on how closely their recall matched the events in the film (20 = completely accurate, 0 = not at all accurate).

The results of the experiment are shown in Table 1.

Table 1: The median accuracy score for the standard interview and the cognitive interview.

	Standard interview	*Cognitive interview*
Median	10	15

The experiment used an independent groups design. Explain how this study could have been modified by using a matched pairs design. [4 marks]

The researcher needs to ensure that the two groups are matched for key variables, such as eyesight, age and intelligence. These variables may affect memory in this situation. All participants should be tested beforehand as regards these variables. Finally, for each person in one condition, the researcher should assign a 'matched' person in the other condition. (56 words)

02 Identify and outline two techniques that may be used in a cognitive interview. [4 marks]

Changing perspective – the interviewee recalls from different perspectives e.g. how it would have appeared to other witnesses.
Report everything – the interviewer encourages the interviewee to recall and report everything they remember, even though it may seem irrelevant. (37 words)

0 3 *Outline and evaluate research into the effects of leading questions on the accuracy of eyewitness testimony.* [8 marks]

Loftus and Palmer conducted studies into eyewitness testimony in 1974. They played a video of a car crash to participants and asked them 'how fast was the car going when it...the other car'. In different conditions they found that if they used the word 'smashed' the participants estimated an average speed of 41 miles per hour compared to an average estimation of 32 miles per hour if they used the word 'contacted'. A week later they also asked 'Did you see any broken glass?' using the word 'smashed' for one group, 'hit' for another and a third control group had no indication of speed given to them. The 'smashed' group had a higher number reporting 'broken glass', even though there was none.

In evaluating, we are aware that viewing a car crash on video is not as emotionally stimulating and produces less adrenaline than being in a real car crash and this may affect the results as it is also less ecologically valid. The participants may have also guessed the aims of the experiment and thus shown demand characteristics. However, both experiments also show that leading questions may have a long-term effect on eyewitness testimony. (196 words)

Section C
Attachment

0 1 Read the item and then answer the question that follows.

Proud father Abdul was talking to his friend, as they were both watching Abdul's wife, Tasneem, interacting with their baby daughter, Aisha.
'It's amazing really', said Abdul. 'Tasneem smiles, Aisha smiles back. Tasneem moves her head, Aisha moves hers, perfectly in time with each other.'
'Yes', agreed the friend. 'It's almost as if they are one person.'

With reference to Abdul's conversation with his friend, outline two features of caregiver-infant interaction. [4 marks]

Interactional synchrony – infant and adult react and respond in time to sustain communication. This is shown when the friend says, 'It's almost as if they are one person'.
Imitation – infant copies/mimics adult. This is shown when, 'Tasneem smiles, Aisha smiles back.'
(41 words)

0 2 Read the item and then answer the question that follows.

Studies of attachment often involve observation of interactions between mother and baby pairs like Tasneem and Aisha. Researchers sometimes write down everything that happens as it takes place, including their own interpretation of the events.

Explain how such observational research might be refined through the use of behavioural categories. [4 marks]

Clear focus – using categories provides clear focus for the researcher. Categories also enable the proposal of a testable hypothesis. Behavioural categories also allow

observers to tally observations into pre-arranged groupings and to allow for more objective/scientific data recording.
(38 words)

0 3 Read the item and then answer the question that follows.

Joe was taken away from his alcoholic parents at six months old and placed in care. He was adopted when he was seven years old, but has a difficult relationship with his adoptive parents. He is aggressive towards his younger siblings and is often in trouble at school. His last school report said, 'Joe struggles with classwork and seems to have little regard for the feelings of others.'

Discuss Bowlby's maternal deprivation theory. Refer to the experience of Joe as part of your discussion. [12 marks]

Bowlby's maternal deprivation theory could explain why Joe 'has a difficult relationship with his adoptive parents.' This could be because Joe may have formed a single monotropic attachment to his mother until he was 'six months old' which would have been broken when he was 'placed in care'. Bowlby believed in a critical period for forming attachments and as Joe was adopted at 'seven years old' Joe is beyond the critical period for forming attachments. According to Bowlby if attachment is disrupted or not formed during the critical period then an attachment will not be formed.

Joe also appears unable to form secure social bonds, which explains why he is 'aggressive towards his younger siblings.' Bowlby also stated that a consequence of maternal deprivation was a low IQ (Intelligence Quota) which may explain why Joe 'struggles with classwork'. As his critical period was spent in care, Joe's difficult relationships may be due to a lack of opportunity to develop an internal working model. Bowlby stated that the internal working model acted as a template for later relationships. This may mean that Joe is both intellectually and emotionally stunted.

Joe's absence of a monotropic bond and therefore his maternal deprivation could also link to delinquency, according to Bowlby. This is potentially demonstrated as he is 'often in trouble at school' and may have affectionless psychopathy according to Bowlby as he has 'little regard for the feelings of others'. However, some believe that Bowlby overemphasised the role of the mother and monotropy upon a child's development and further to the contrasting views of other psychologists it was Bowlby himself who stated in later years that a monotropic bond could also form securely with the father.

(283 words)

Words: 1698. Copyright: Joseph Campbell 2016.

AQA AS PSYCHOLOGY (7181/1)
PAPER 1
INTRODUCTORY TOPICS IN PSYCHOLOGY.
SPECIMEN MATERIAL SECOND SET

Section A
Social influence

0 1 Many people have criticised Zimbardo's prison study.
Identify and briefly discuss two reasons why people have criticised Zimbardo's prison study. [6 marks]

Two reasons that people have criticised Zimbardo's prison study are for the reasons that they believed it to be unethical as it led to psychological harm as the participants soon became distressed and for the fact that Zimbardo himself took part in the experiment and was a participant observer.

The distress of the participants should have been anticipated beforehand and informed consent should have been gained before the experiment began. Zimbardo caused the participants to have emotional distress and the participants appeared unaware at times of their right to withdraw. Zimbardo also acted as the prison superintendent in this experiment which could lead to observer bias and demonstrates a clear conflict of interests. Thus, the overall validity of the findings themselves could be questioned.
(124 words)

0 2 Social influence research helps us to understand how it is possible to change people's behaviour: for example, understanding how to persuade people to eat more healthily.
With reference to this example of social change, explain how psychology might affect the economy. [4 marks]

Social influence research informs us how both behaviour and attitudes can be changed. For example, how minority influence can be exerted or how people tend to conform to perceived norms. In the example listed above, the resulting change of eating more healthily leads to an increase in the general health of these people. This has an economic implication and saves health services and care resources and potentially increases economic production through less people taking time off work.
(77 words)

0 3 Read the item and then answer the question that follows.

Polly always checks what her friends are going to wear before she gets ready to go out because she does not like to be the odd one out. Jed watches his colleagues carefully when he starts a new job so that he can work out where to put his things and how long to take for lunch.

Discuss two explanations for conformity. Refer to Polly and Jed in your discussion. [12 marks]

Normative social influence occurs when people conform in order to be a part of the majority and to not stand out. Normative social influence often, but not always, results in compliance or a superficial change in behaviour. Informational social influence occurs when people conform in order to be fully aware as to how to behave in a given situation and therefore use the majority as a source of information. This often results in internalisation i.e. adopting the views and behaviours of the majority.

Polly's behaviour is due to normative social influence because she desires to be the same as everyone else and to be a part of the 'norm'. Jed is using his colleagues as a source of information which is informational social influence. He will learn 'where to put his things' and take the appropriate amount of time for lunch.

Informational social influence tends to have a more permanent effect whereas normative social influence tends to be more transient. There is also the possibility of an overlap between the two types of social influence as we often look to others for information but partly because we do not want to be different.

In Asch's (1951) study upon conformity as regards an unambiguous task, 37% were wrong and conformed to the majority due to normative social influence. However different conditions of the study illustrated both normative and informational social influence supporting the idea of an overlap between these two explanations of conformity.

(242 words)

Section B
Memory

0 1 Read the item and then answer the questions that follow.

A researcher investigating the multi-store model of memory tested short-term memory by reading out loud sequences of numbers that participants then had to repeat aloud immediately after presentation. The first sequence was made up of three numbers: for example, 8, 5, 2. Each participant was tested several times, and each time the length of the sequence was increased by adding another number.

Use your knowledge of the multi-store model of memory to explain the purpose of this research and the likely outcome. [4 marks]

The purpose of this research is to test the capacity of short-term memory. Short-term memories are coded both verbally and acoustically and this research requires verbal rehearsal. The outcome would most likely be that most of the people tested would be able to repeat correctly a sequence of between 5 and 9 items. This is because according to the multi-store model, short-term memory has a limited capacity of between 5 and 9 items. (73 words)

0 2 After the study was completed, the researcher decided to modify the study by using sequences of letters rather than numbers.

Suggest one 4-letter sequence and one 5-letter sequence that the researcher could use. In the case of each sequence, give a justification for your choice. Use a different justification for each sequence. [4 marks]

ZXLM is the appropriate 4-letter sequence I would suggest. This is because it has no recognisable abbreviations which have meaning and can be recalled as a whole.

JXFKD is the appropriate 5-letter sequence I would suggest. This is because it has no rhyming letters, which would mean that the cognitive demand would be reduced for the participants and could influence the research (if it contained rhyming letters). (67 words)

0 3 *Read the item and then answer the question that follows.*

Martin is studying for his modern language exams. He revises French followed by Spanish on the same night and then gets confused between the two: for example, he remembers the French word for 'chair' instead of the Spanish word for 'chair'. Sometimes, his mum helps to test Martin's vocabulary. When he is unable to remember a word, his mum tells him the first letter, then he can often recall it correctly.

Discuss two explanations for forgetting. Refer to Martin's experiences in your answer. [12 marks]

Interference is an explanation for forgetting as two sets of information can become confused, such as Spanish and French in Martin's case when he gets confused between the two. There are two types of interference; proactive interference and retroactive interference. Proactive interference is when old learning prevents the recall of more recent information, shown when Martin 'remembers the French word for 'chair' instead of the Spanish word for 'chair'' as Martin 'revises French followed by Spanish'. Retroactive interference is when new learning prevents the recall of previously learned information. As French and Spanish are similar types of material this makes interference more likely. There is a question as to whether interference involves the over-writing of other information and it is said that semantic memory is more resistant to interference than other types of memory.

Retrieval failure which is also known as cue-dependent forgetting has also been posited as an explanation for forgetting. This is demonstrated when information is available but cannot be recalled because of the absence of appropriate cues. The types of cues that have been studied by psychologists include context, state and organisation. Cues improve recall if recall takes place in the same context as learning, if the person is in the same physical state as when the material was learned and if triggers or categories are assigned in order to achieve cue-dependent learning. For example, Martin's mum gives him cues, 'tells him the first letter' which can then be used for him to access the material he has failed to retrieve.

Both explanations for forgetting have general implications for both revision and other situations.

(267 words)

By Joseph Anthony Campbell

Section C
Attachment

0 1 Read the item and then answer the questions that follow.

A child psychologist carried out an overt observation of caregiver-infant interaction. She observed a baby boy interacting separately with each of his parents. Using a time sampling technique, she observed the baby with each parent for 10 minutes. Her findings are shown in Table 1 below.

Table 1: Frequency of each behaviour displayed by the infant when interacting with his mother and when interacting with his father

	Gazing at parent	Looking away from parent	Eyes closed	Total
Mother	12	2	6	20
Father	6	10	4	20
Total	18	12	10	40

Using the data in Table 1, explain the procedure used for the time sampling technique in this study. [3 marks]

The total observation time for each parent was 10 minutes. The psychologist made 20 observations for each parent. To generate 20 observations for each parent she must therefore have recorded her observation every 30 seconds. (35 words)

0 2 In what percentage of the total observations was the baby gazing at his mother? Show your calculations. [2 marks]

12 / 40 = 0.3
0.3 x 100 = 30%
Answer = 30%

0 3 The study in Question 09 was an overt observation. Explain what is meant by 'overt observation'. [2 marks]

Overt observation is when the observer is clearly visible and not hidden from view. Also, the people being observed know that they are being observed. (25 words)

0 4 Outline the procedure used in one study of animal attachment. [4 marks]

Harlow aimed to find out whether baby rhesus monkeys would prefer a source of food or a source of comfort and protection as an attachment figure. In laboratory experiments the rhesus monkeys were raised in isolation. They had two 'surrogate' mothers. One was made of wire mesh and contained a feeding bottle; the other was made of cloth but didn't contain a feeding bottle. (64 words)

0 5 Briefly discuss one limitation of using animals to study attachment in humans. [4 marks]

There are problems of extrapolation in applying the results to human infants. What applies to non-human species may not also apply to human infants. For example, Lorenz studied imprinting in geese, which are a precocial species i.e. they have their eyes open and walk from birth. This is very different to humans who cannot walk for a few years. Therefore, attachment studies using animals should be studied carefully. (68 words)

0 6 One theory about how and why babies form attachments is Bowlby's monotropic theory. Outline and evaluate Bowlby's monotropic theory of attachment [8 marks]

According to Bowlby we have evolved a biological need to attach to our main caregiver. His idea is called monotropy and it states that we form one main attachment, usually to our biological mother. This attachment has survival value as staying close to our mother ensures food and protection. It also gives us a 'template' for all future relationships as we learn to trust and care for others. This forms an internal working model for all later attachments. The first three years of life are posited by Bowlby as the 'critical period' for attachment to develop or it may never do so.

However, Schaffer et al provided evidence against Bowlby's theory. They found that many children form multiple attachments and may not attach to their mother. This contrasts with Bowlby's theory of monotropy. Also, in Harlow's study other monkeys who did not have a primary caregiver but grew up together, seemed to attach to each other instead and showed no signs of social or emotional disturbance in later life. (169 words)

Words: 1884. Copyright: Joseph Campbell 2016.

AQA AS PSYCHOLOGY (7181/2)
PAPER 2
PSYCHOLOGY IN CONTEXT
SPECIMEN MATERIAL (FIRST SET)

Section A
Approaches in Psychology

0 1 *Read the item and then answer the question that follows.*

Psychologists investigating theoretical models of cognitive processing study human cognitive processing. They sometimes give participants problems to solve then ask them about the experience afterwards. Typical participant responses are as follows:
Response A: 'There were too many things to think about at the same time.'
Response B: 'I had to do one task at a time, then do the next task, and so on.'

Briefly suggest how each of these responses might inform psychologists investigating models of human cognitive processing. [2 marks]

Response A shows that processing has limited capacity and response B demonstrates that in order for a participant to complete demanding or new processes they must do them sequentially.

0 2 *Read the item and then answer the questions that follow.*

A behaviourist researcher studying reinforcement carried out a laboratory experiment. He put a cat in a puzzle box. The cat was able to escape from the puzzle box by pulling on a string which opened the door. Each time the cat escaped it was given a food treat. At first, the cat escaped quite slowly, but with each attempt the escape time decreased.

Explain which type of conditioning is being investigated in this experiment? [2 marks]

Operant conditioning is being investigated in this experiment as the cat is rewarded with food to positively reinforce certain behaviour, in this case 'pulling the string'.

0 3 Read the item and then answer the questions that follow.

A psychologist carried out a study of social learning. As part of the procedure, he showed children aged 4-5 years a film of a 4-year-old boy stroking a puppy. Whilst the children watched the film, the psychologist commented on how kind the boy was. After the children had watched the film, the psychologist brought a puppy into the room and watched to see how the children behaved with the puppy.

Outline what is meant by social learning theory and explain how social learning might have occurred in the procedure described above. [6 marks]

Social learning theory states that individuals can learn from role models. An individual may observe and imitate and therefore model themselves on another person. This is known as modelling. This role model must be someone that the person can identify with e.g. they are of a similar age or the same gender. Social leaning theory approach (SLT) states that behaviour can also be taught through positive and negative reinforcement and vicarious reinforcement (seeing others being rewarded for certain behaviours). For effective learning, meditational processes must also take place, such as attention which involves an attentional focus on the behaviour being copied and reproduction which involves judging whether you are able to imitate the behaviour observed.

In this experiment SLT is taking place as the psychologist provided the children with a role model the same age as them acting pro-socially by 'stroking a puppy.' The children were also encouraged to identify with the role model and this makes them highly likely to imitate him. This acted as vicarious reinforcement and the children may imitate his behaviour in the hope of being praised although some may not perform these actions due to the internalisation of the model not being visibly manifested immediately.

0 4 Discuss two limitations of social learning theory. [6 marks]

Social learning theory posits that behaviours are learnt from the environment and this does not explain how some behaviours appear to be innate such as reflexes. Furthermore, SLT is unable to explain abstract notions such as justice or fairness. It explains the learning of outward behaviours but not abstract notions which are less simplistic and which cannot be observed directly.

Psychologists are also unable to establish cause and effect when studying SLT. This is because SLT may not produce outward behaviours at the time that the original learning took place. It may be a significant period of time before these observed behaviours are internalised and thus manifested. Although Bandura's research-controlled variables and had replicable results it is still difficult to establish this cause and effect in real life.

Section B
Psychopathology

0 1 Read the item and then answer the questions that follow.

Researchers analysed the behaviour of over 4000 pairs of twins. The results showed that the degree to which obsessive-compulsive disorder (OCD) is inherited is between 45% and 65%.

Distinguish between obsessions and compulsions. [2 marks]

Obsessions are intrusive and persistent thoughts that can lead someone to act upon their compulsions. These compulsions are actions such as obsessive hand washing that temporarily reduce the anxiety of the obsessive thoughts. (33 words)

0 2 With reference to the study described above, what do the results seem to show about possible influences on the development of OCD? [4 marks]

This study demonstrates that obsessive-compulsive disorder (OCD) may/does have a genetic basis. This is shown as between 45% to 65% of OCD is inherited, which supports a biological basis for the development of OCD.
However, there is still 35% to 55% of OCD that is not inherited, showing that there must be other components to the development of OCD such as cognitive and behavioural abnormalities. (65 words)

0 3 Read the item and then answer the question that follows.

Steven describes how he feels when he is in a public place. 'I always have to look out for people who might be ill. If I come into contact with people who look ill, I think I might catch it and die. If someone starts to cough or sneeze then I have to get away and clean myself quickly.'

Outline one cognitive characteristic of OCD and one behavioural characteristic of OCD that can be identified from the description provided by Steven. [2 marks]

A cognitive characteristic is that Steven had obsessive thoughts e.g. he always has 'to look out for people who might be ill'. This is also known as hyper vigilance.

A behavioural characteristic is the compulsion that Steven has that he must 'get away and clean myself quickly' if someone sneezes or coughs. (52 words)

0 4 Briefly outline one strength of the cognitive explanation of depression. [2 marks]

The cognitive explanation of depression takes into account the thoughts and beliefs of an individual and this has led to reasonably effective treatments for depression as it is based on sound experimental research. (33 words)

0 5 Outline and evaluate the behavioural approach to treating phobias. [12 marks]

The behavioural approach to treating phobias consists of systematic desensitisation and flooding. Flooding consists of putting an individual into a place or a scenario or into a visualisation of their set phobia i.e. such as arachnophobia- the fear of spiders. This would trigger their phobia immediately and they would be left to face their phobia until their anxiety levels decline and their phobia is eliminated. This method is immediate and fairly cheap leading to more accessibility for people to eliminate their phobia. However, some argue that it is unethical as it causes the patient emotional distress. Also, if they leave before their phobia is fully extinguished it can heighten or worsen their phobic levels.

Systematic desensitisation involves gradually working up a patients fear hierarchy until the patient is able to maintain a relaxed state when confronted with the situation that triggers their phobia the most such as holding a spider if arachnophobic. As the patient moves upwards on the hierarchical scale, they may have their treatment initiated by simply viewing a picture of a spider. The patient is taught relaxation techniques beforehand such as deep breathing in order to apply these techniques as their anxiety is triggered whilst moving up the fear hierarchy. Systematic desensitisation uses counter-conditioning which results in the patient no longer associating the stimulus with danger and thus anxiety.

Zinbarg et al (1992) found that systematic desensitisation was the most effective of all contemporary treatments and Ost et al found that 90% of patients experienced anxiety reduction after just one session in both flooding and systematic desensitisation. Behavioural therapy also treats symptoms rather than cognitive behavioural therapy which focuses more on the causes of anxiety.

(278 words)

Section C
Research methods

0 1 *Read the item and then answer the questions that follow.*

A psychologist wanted to see if creativity is affected by the presence of other people. To test this, he arranged for 30 people to participate in a study that involved generating ideas for raising funds for a local youth club. Participants were randomly allocated to one of two conditions.

Condition A: there were 15 participants in this condition. Each participant was placed separately in a room and was given 40 minutes to think of as many ideas as possible for raising funds for a local youth club. The participant was told to write down his or her ideas and these were collected in by the psychologist at the end of the 40 minutes.

Condition B: there were 15 participants in this condition. The participants were randomly allocated to 5 groups of equal size. Each group was given 40 minutes to think of as many ideas as possible for raising funds for a local youth club. Each group was told to write down their ideas and these were collected by the psychologist at the end of the 40 minutes.

The psychologist counted the number of ideas generated by the participants in both conditions and calculated the total number of ideas for each condition.

Table 2: Total number of ideas generated in Condition A (when working alone) and in Condition B (when working in a group)

	Condition A Working alone	Condition B Working in a group
Total number of ideas generated	110	75

Identify the experimental design used in this study and outline one advantage of this experimental design. [3 marks]

The experimental design used is an independent groups design; an advantage of this is that there are no order effects. This means that no participant improves with practice i.e. learning effect or has their performance negatively affected by fatigue effect.

0 2 Describe one other experimental design that researchers use in psychology. [2 marks]

Another experimental design used is a repeated measures design. This is when all the participants participate in all the conditions.

0 3 Apart from using random allocation, suggest one way in which the psychologist might have improved this study by controlling for the effects of extraneous variables. Justify your answer. [2 marks]

The psychologist could have tested all of the participants in the same room as this would ensure that participants will not receive cues from their surroundings and that extraneous variables will not interfere with the experiment's findings.

0 4 Write a suitable hypothesis for this study. [3 marks]

Those participants that work on their own and those that work in groups are equally likely to generate ideas. (Null hypothesis and non-directional)

0 5 From the information given in the description, calculate the number of participants in each group in Condition B. [1 mark]

15/5 = 3

0 6 Read the item and then answer the questions that follow.

The psychologist noticed that the number of ideas generated by each of the individual participants in Condition A varied enormously whereas there was little variation in performance between the 5 groups in Condition B. He decided to calculate a measure of dispersion for each condition.

Name a measure of dispersion the psychologist could use. [1 mark]

Standard deviation.

0 7 *The psychologist uses the measure of dispersion you have named in your answer to question o 6. State how the result for each condition would differ. [1 mark]*

The standard deviation would be greater in condition A than in condition B.

0 8 Explain how the psychologist could have used random allocation to assign the 15 participants in Condition B into the 5 groups. [3 marks]

The psychologist could have numbered the participants between 1 and 15. He could then put the 15 numbers in a hat. He could then draw out 3 numbers to create the first group and repeat the process until all participants are in five groups of 3.

0 9 Using the information given, explain how the psychologist could further analyse the data using percentages. [2 marks]

The psychologist would add the total number of ideas generated in both conditions which is 185. The psychologist then divides each condition by 185 and multiplies this by 100 to receive the percentage.

1 0 At the end of the study the psychologist debriefed each participant. Write a debriefing that the psychologist could read out to the participants in Condition A. [6 marks]

The aim of this experiment is to discern whether working in groups affected the number of ideas generated in comparison to working alone. The study consisted of two conditions of which you would have been assigned to either condition A or condition B. Condition A consisted of one person generating ideas and condition B consisted of a group generating ideas.

You will be informed of the results at a later date and your data will be kept wholly anonymous. Your welfare is of vital importance and if you have any questions or ethical concerns please feel free to talk to the researcher. You retain the right to withdraw at this point and we wish to thank you for taking part in this experiment. We hope it has been a worthwhile experience for you.

Words: 2251. Copyright: Joseph Campbell 2016.

AQA AS PSYCHOLOGY (7181/2)
PAPER 2
PSYCHOLOGY IN CONTEXT
SPECIMEN MATERIAL (SECOND SET)

Section A
Approaches in Psychology

0 1 *Briefly explain one function of the endocrine system. [2 marks]*

The endocrine system involves glands which secrete hormones. The adrenal gland produces the hormone adrenaline which is responsible for our 'fight or flight (or freeze)' reaction when we are stressed.

0 2 *A cognitive psychologist investigating how memory works gave participants the same word list to recall in one of two conditions. All the words were of equal difficulty.*

Condition 1: Ten participants recalled the words in the same room in which they had learned the words.

Condition 2: Ten different participants recalled the words in a room that was not the same room as that in which they had learned the words.

The following results were obtained:

Table 1: Mean values and standard deviations for Condition 1 and Condition 2 in a memory experiment.

	Condition 1	Condition 2
Mean	15.9	10.6
Standard deviation	3.78	1.04

Why are the standard deviation values found in the study above useful descriptive statistics for the cognitive psychologist? [2 marks]

Standard deviation values show a spread of scores and the range and delineate participant variables (condition 1 indicates there were more variables than condition 2).

0 3 Outline one problem of studying internal mental processes like memory ability by conducting experiments such as that described in Question 03 above. [2 marks]

In an internal mental process, the researcher is unable to observe the process. This provides a problem as the researcher has to infer what processes are taking place by the behaviour the participant exhibits and this can easily lead to errors.

0 4 Rita and Holly are identical twins who were separated at birth. When they finally met each other at the age of 35, they were surprised at how different their personalities were. Rita is much more social and out-going than Holly.

Use your knowledge of genotype and phenotype to explain this difference in their personalities. [4 marks]

As Rita and Holly are monozygotic twins their genotypes are the same. This means that genetically they carry the same genetic predispositions. However, it is possible that external factors may contribute to their development also such as differing environments and this could begin to explain why Rita and Holly have such different phenotypes. The difference in phenotypes may be due to Rita being placed in situations were being sociable was rewarded whilst Holly was not.

0 5 Outline and evaluate the social learning theory approach. Refer to evidence in your answer. [12 marks]

Social learning theory states that individuals can learn from role models. An individual may observe and imitate and therefore model themselves on another person. This is known as modelling. This role model must be someone that the person can identify with e.g. they are of a similar age or the same gender. Social leaning theory approach (SLT) states that behaviour can also be taught through positive and negative reinforcement and vicarious reinforcement (seeing others being rewarded for certain behaviours). For effective learning, meditational processes must also take place, such as attention which involves an attentional focus on the behaviour being copied and reproduction which involves judging whether you are able to imitate the behaviour observed.

There is evidence to support SLT such as Bandura's study on the imitation of aggression. This study showed that children who were exposed to aggressive models tend to imitate the aggressive model's behaviour. However, because the learning is internalised and the learning could take place long before the behaviour is exhibited, it is hard to establish cause and effect when studying SLT. SLT is also reductionist and fails to take into account any other explanations for learning such as biological or genetic influences. SLT also does not explain the cognitive processes that cause an individual to want to copy a role model or certain behaviours that they demonstrate. SLT does however explain human traits which the behavioural approach neglects.

Section B
Psychopathology

0 1 What is meant by 'statistical infrequency' as a definition of abnormality? [2 marks]

This is when an individual's traits widely differ to that of the average population. It is when they fall either side of a bell curve of the population on a graph for example if an individual's intelligence quota (IQ) was 150 and the average populations was 100. (47 words)

0 2 Gavin describes his daily life.

'I sometimes get gripped with the thought that my family is in danger. In particular, I worry about them being trapped in a house fire. I now find that I can only calm myself if I check that every plug socket is switched off so an electrical fire couldn't start. I used to switch each socket on and off, but now I have to press each switch six times. It takes me ages to leave the house.'

Outline two characteristics of obsessive-compulsive disorder. Refer to Gavin in your answer. [4 marks]

Gavin has persistent and recurring thoughts which are characteristic of the obsessive component of obsessive-compulsive disorder (OCD). An example of this is shown when he states, 'I sometimes get gripped with the thought that my family is in danger'. Gavin also has compulsions shown through partaking in repetitive actions that temporarily reduce the anxiety caused by the obsessions. Gavin has to 'press each switch six times' in order to calm his obsessions. This is characteristic of OCD. (77 words)

0 3 Read the item and then answer the question that follows.

Tommy is six years old and has a phobia about birds. His mother is worried because he now refuses to go outside. She says, 'Tommy used to love playing in the garden and going to the park to play football with his friends, but he is spending more and more time watching TV and on the computer.'

A psychologist has suggested treating Tommy's fear of birds using systematic desensitisation. Explain how this procedure could be used to help Tommy overcome his phobia. [4 marks]

Tommy would be taught relaxation techniques, such as deep breathing. Tommy would then devise a fear hierarchy with the situation that triggers his phobia the most at the top of the fear hierarchy such as holding a bird and the situation that triggers his phobia the least at the bottom of the hierarchical scale such as looking at a picture of a bird. Tommy would then work his way up the fear hierarchy by being exposed to his phobia of birds gradually and move up to the next item on the hierarchical scale when he is no longer anxious with a set stage. If his anxiety increases the psychologist would guide him to a lower stage on the hierarchical scale. Tommy could also use the relaxation techniques he has previously learned to calm himself down. Eventually Tommy may be able to fully overcome his phobia. (145 words)

0 4 Explain why systematic desensitisation might be more ethical than using flooding to treat Tommy's phobia. [2 marks]

Flooding involves making a person confront their phobia fully until their anxiety has worn off. However, Tommy's anxiety levels may increase dramatically though flooding whilst systematic desensitisation is more gradual and limits the levels of anxiety experienced by the participant. (40 words)

0 5 Outline and evaluate at least one cognitive approach to explaining depression. [12 marks]

Ellis' ABC model posits that depression originates with an activating event such as the break-up of a relationship which then leads to an irrational belief such as 'I am unlovable'. This belief results in a consequence which may lead to depression.

Beck's negative triad posits that a person is depressed because they have negative thoughts about themselves (I am unlovable), the world (no one will ever love me because I am unlovable) and the future (this will continue forever).

The cognitive models above offer a useful approach to explaining depression as thoughts and feelings are taken into account. Cognitive behavioural therapies have also successfully treated depression. Psychologists have also demonstrated that depressed participants have more negative thoughts than non-depressed participants and this demonstrates a clear correlation between depression and negative thinking.

However, faulty cognitions may be a symptom or consequence of depression rather than the cause. The person may have a biological abnormality that causes negative thinking. This theory also is reductionist as it reduces complex human phenomena into simplistic human terminology and it does not take into account both behavioural and biological influences. (184 words)

Section C
Research Methods

Read the item and then answer the questions that follow.

Two researchers obtained a sample of ten people whose ages ranged from 20-years-old to 60-years-old.

Each participant was asked to take part in a discussion of social care issues. This included discussion about who should pay for social care for elderly people and how to deal with people struggling with mental health problems. A confederate of the researchers was given a script to follow in which a series of discussion points was written for the confederate to introduce.

Each participant then came into a room individually and the discussion with the confederate took place. The maximum time allowed for a discussion was 30 minutes.

The researchers observed the discussions between the confederate and participants and rated the active engagement of the participants in the discussion. The ratings were between 1, (not at all interested) and 20, (extremely interested.) The researchers believed that the rating provided a measurement of the participants' attitudes towards social care issues.

The following data were obtained in the study:

Table 2: The relationship between age and attitude to social care

Age of participant	Attitude to social care issues rating
21	5
23	3
34	8
36	12
40	10

47	13
52	17
53	15
58	18
60	20

0 1 What does the table suggest about the relationship between age and attitude to social care issues? Explain your answer. [2 marks]

The table suggests a positive correlation between the age of the participant and their attitude to social care issues. The relationship between age and attitude to social care issues shows that as the age of the participant increases so does their attitude to social care issues rating generally.

0 2 The researchers rated the active engagement of the participants in the discussion on social care. They used this rating as a measure of each participant's attitude to social care issues. Briefly explain how investigator effects might have occurred in this study. [2 marks]

The investigator effect is when the investigator has knowledge of the research aim and this knowledge affects the data collected. This can affect results as the experimenter may have preconceived ideas as to how age affects our levels of interest in social care issues.

0 3 Outline how the researchers could have avoided investigator effects having an impact on the study. [2 marks]

Investigator effects could have been nullified by having two researchers assess the group discussion and comparing their scores to see if they match or are similar. This is known as inter-rater reliability.

0 4 The researchers thought it might be interesting to investigate further the attitudes of the participants in the study. They decided to interview each participant. The researchers devised a questionnaire in order to collect the data they required. The questionnaire included both open and closed questions.

Briefly discuss the benefits for the researchers of using both closed and open questions on their questionnaire about attitudes to social care. [4 marks]

Closed questions enable researchers to obtain quantitative data (facts, figures, known as hard data etc.) which is easier to analyse and draw conclusions from. However closed questions may not obtain important data from the participants as closed questions only collect data that the researchers believe to be relevant.

Open questions collect qualitative data (thoughts, feelings, known as soft data etc.) which is harder to analyse and draw clear cut conclusions from. However open questions enable the researchers to have the participants expand upon their answers.

0 5 Write one question that you think the researchers might have put on their questionnaire. Explain which type of question you have written and why you think this would be a suitable question for this study. [3 marks]

'Have you researched the types of social care that are available in this country?' This is a closed question and thus enables the researcher to collect quantitative data which is easier to analyse than qualitative data.

0 6 The researchers have obtained both qualitative and quantitative data in the observations and interviews they have conducted.

Identify the qualitative and quantitative data collected in this study. Explain your answer. [4 marks]

Quantitative data is collected from closed questions and will be numerically based, facts, figures etc. and is sometimes known as hard data i.e. a score represented in the form of a score on a scale.

Qualitative data is collected from open questions and is descriptive of thoughts, feelings and emotions etc. and could be found in the attitude's ratings.

0 7 Explain how the researchers should have addressed two ethical issues in the investigation. [4 marks]

The right to withdraw should be made clear to the participants so that they are clearly aware that they can withdraw from the experiment at any time without facing negative consequences.

Informed consent should also be obtained and the participants should be forewarned of what the experiment will entail and be briefed and debriefed and they should also be given clear information as to what the investigation will involve.

Words: 2265. Copyright: Joseph Campbell 2016.

AQA A-LEVEL PSYCHOLOGY (7182/1)
PAPER 1
INTRODUCTORY TOPICS IN PSYCHOLOGY.
SPECIMEN MATERIAL
2017
HTTP://FILESTORE.AQA.ORG.UK/RESOURCES/PSYCHOLOGY/AQA-71821-SQP.PDF

Section A
Social influence

Answer **all** questions in this section

0 1 Which of the following terms best matches the statements below? Choose **one** term that matches **each** statement and write A, B, C, D or E in the box next to it. Use each letter once only.

A Identification
B Informational social influence
C Normative social influence
D Compliance
E Internalisation

Publicly changing behaviour whilst maintaining a different private view. [1 mark]
D

Group pressure leading to a desire to fit in with the group. [1 mark]
C

When a person lacks knowledge of how to behave and looks to the group for guidance. [1 mark]
B

Conforming to the behaviour of a role model. [1 mark]
A

*0 2 Briefly outline **and** evaluate the findings of any **one** study of social influence. [4 marks]*

Asch placed male participants in an unambiguous situation where the majority of participants conformed at least once when confederates gave the same wrong answer to a question comparing line lengths across various trials. 75% of participants conformed at least once across 18 trials.

The study lacks ecological validity however, as whether the participants were right or wrong did not really matter to the participants; they may have been less likely to conform if their answers had real-life consequences. Also, in terms of ethics, the participants were deceived as to the true nature of the study.

0 3 Read the item and then answer the question that follows.

Two psychology students were discussing the topic of social influence.
'I find it fascinating how some people are able to resist social influence', said Jack. 'It must be the result of having a confident personality.'
'I disagree', replied Sarah. 'I think resisting social influence depends much more on the presence of others.'
*Discuss **two** explanations of resistance to social influence. As part of your discussion, refer to the views expressed by Jack and Sarah in the conversation above. [16 marks]*

One explanation of resistance to social influence is that of social support, a situational factor. Sarah states that resistance depends on 'the presence of others' and Milgram found that participants are less likely to obey authority if there were other dissenting confederates present. Asch found similar results in variations of his experiment on conformity in an unambiguous situation when he tested the effect of the participant having a supporter in the group. Instead of the confederates forming a unanimous majority, one of the confederates agreed with the participant. Having a fellow dissenter who disagreed with the majority broke the unanimity of the group. This made it easier for the participant to resist the pressure to conform and the rate of conformity fell to 5.5%. This finding is reflected in Sarah's comment that 'social influence depends much more on the presence of others.' This explanation of resistance to social influence provides a viable explanation through a situational factor as to why people would resist social influence.

Jack however suggests that dispositional factors in resisting social influence are more important. Another explanation of resistance is that of 'locus of control'. Jack states that '…how some people are able to resist social influence…must be the result of having a confident personality'. If someone has an internal locus of control, they are more likely to accept personal responsibility for their own actions. They are therefore less likely to obey authoritative demands that are against both their morals and views. If someone has an external locus of control, they are less likely to accept personal responsibility for their actions and are therefore more likely to feel helpless and obedient when confronted with a perceived authority figure. This explanation of resistance to social influence provides an alternative, viable explanation through a dispositional factor as to why people would resist social influence.

However as to the psychological experiments that have provided these two explanations of resistance to social influence, both Asch and Milgram's experiments have been criticised for the deceptive elements of their studies. Asch and Milgram' participants encounter the ethical issue of deception as Asch's participants believed that they were taking part in a study to determine line lengths whilst Milgram's participants believed that the experiment was based on the effects of punishment on learning and that they were actually providing electric shocks to participants. The experiments could have had a long-term impact on the participants and both experiments could therefore lack validity and be criticised for their levels of ecological validity due to the fact that they were both artificial laboratory experiments.

Section B
Memory

Answer **all** questions in this section

Read the item and then answer the questions that follow.

An experiment was carried out to test the effects of learning similar and dissimilar information on participants' ability to remember.

In **Stage 1** of the experiment, 10 participants in **Group A**, the 'similar' condition, were given a list of 20 place names in the UK. They were given two minutes to learn the list. 10 different participants in **Group B**, the 'dissimilar' condition, were given the same list of 20 place names in the UK. They were also given two minutes to learn the list.

In **Stage 2** of the experiment, participants in **Group A** were given a different list of 20 more place names in the UK, and were given a further two minutes to learn it. Participants in **Group B** were given a list of 20 boys' names, and were given a further two minutes to learn it.

In **Stage 3** of the experiment, all participants were given five minutes to recall as many of the 20 place names in the UK, from the list in **Stage 1**, as they could. The raw data from the two groups is below.

Table 1: Number of place names recalled from the list in Stage 1.

Group A	Group B
5	11
6	10
4	11
7	13
8	12
4	14
5	15
4	11
6	14
7	14

0 4-0 1 *What is the most appropriate measure of central tendency for calculating the average of the scores, from **Table 1**, in each of the **two** groups? Justify your answer. [2 marks]*

The mean is the appropriate measure of central tendency for calculating the average of the scores. The mean is the most sensitive method as it takes all the scores in each data set into account. (35 words)

0 4-0 2 *Calculate the measure of central tendency you have identified in your answer to **question 04.0 1** for **Group A** and **Group B**. Show your calculations for each group. [4 marks]*

5+6+4+7+8+4+5+4+6+7=56/10= 5.6 = Group A mean
11+10+11+13+12+14+15+11+14+14=125/10= 12.5 =Group B mean

0 4-0 3 *In **Stage 3** of the experiment, several participants in **Group A**, the 'similar' condition, recalled words from the **Stage 2** list rather than the **Stage 1** list.*

Use your knowledge of forgetting to explain why this may have occurred. [2 marks]

The information presented in Stage 1 and Stage 2 was similar and the new information disrupted/interfered with the recall of previous information. This is called retroactive interference. (27 words)

0 5 *Describe **and** evaluate the working memory model of memory. [16 marks]*

The working memory model (WMM) was created by Baddeley and Hitch in 1974 and the model proposed that short term memory was comprised of three different stores; the phonological loop, the episodic buffer and the visuo-spatial sketchpad. The central executive receives all of the information that is paid attention to (attentional focus) and directs the information to one of the three slave systems according to its type. Speech-based information is directed to the phonological loop; visual and spatial information is directed towards the visuo-spatial sketchpad and the episodic buffer (2000) stores information from the other two slave systems and integrates the information together to form episodes along with information from long term memory (LTM) in order to make complete scenes or form 'episodes'. All of the slave systems have limited capacity and duration and therefore in order to store information for a long time, information must be passed on to the long-term memory.

The working memory model is supported by evidence such as the case study of KF by Shallice and Washington (1974). KF sustained brain damage in a motorbike accident and had problems with certain areas of short-term memory. KF could recall and process visual information but had trouble recalling words verbally. This suggests that he had an impaired articulatory loop but an intact visuo-spatial sketchpad. KF's condition could not be explained by the multi-store model of memory (MSM) which delineates short term memory as one store and in the case of KF it instead supports the working memory model's theory that short term memory is made up of multiple stores and an active processor unlike the multi-store model of memory which contains a discrete store only.

The working memory model also does not place as much emphasis on rehearsal as the multi-store model. Rehearsal is only one possible process in the working memory model which helps to explain how information enters the long-term memory after little or no rehearsal. This means that the working memory model allows for other explanations on processes rather than one finite explanation as provided by the multi-store model.

However, some psychologists argue that the central executive is too vague and simplistic in its description. They argue that the central executive is a blanket term to describe many processes and stores and that it is merely described as 'attention' in the working memory model. The idea of a central executive is also not supported by evidence as it is extremely difficult to design tasks to test it and therefore there is little empirical evidence.

(422 words)

Section C
Attachment

Answer **all** questions in this section

06 Name **three** stages in the development of attachments identified by Schaffer. *[3 marks]*

1 Pre-attachment
2 Indiscriminate (Multiple)
3 Discriminate

07 Read the item and then answer the question that follows.

A nursery school worker and her manager were chatting at the end of the day.
'How did the new toddlers settle in today?' asked the manager.
'They behaved very differently', replied the nursery school worker. 'Max was distressed when his mother left but was happy to see her at the end of the day.'
'Jessica arrived clinging to her mother and I could not calm her down when her mother left.'
'William barely seemed to notice when his mother left and did not even look up when she returned to collect him.'
*Name the attachment type demonstrated by **each** of the children in the conversation above by writing the attachment type next to the name below. [3 marks]*

Max	Secure
Jessica	Insecure - resistant
William	Insecure - avoidant

0 8 *Briefly evaluate learning theory as an explanation of attachment. [4 marks]*

There is support for the learning theory as an explanation of attachment. Much of the evidence is derived from scientific research involving research on animals. This is a limitation because it presents the problem of anthropomorphic extrapolation because it is not possible to fully extrapolate from animals to humans as humans and animals are inherently different in morals and physicality. It is also difficult to tell in learning theory if an association has taken place and if it ever will take place when studying babies in their early months. Schaffer and Emerson (1964) found that many babies did not have their mother as the primary attachment figure despite the mother being the primary caregiver, in their study. (117 words)

0 9 Read the item and then answer the question that follows.

A group of researchers used 'event sampling' to observe children's friendships over a period of three weeks at break times and lunchtimes during the school day.
Explain what is meant by 'event sampling'. [2 marks]

'Event sampling' is when researchers comprise a list of events they want to study (e.g. holding hands, speaking aloud etc.) and compile a period of time in which to record said events (e.g. 5 hourly periods). The researchers then record the events that occur in the period of time previously designated. (51 words)

1 0 The investigation in **question 09** is an example of a 'naturalistic observation'.
Briefly discuss how observational research might be improved by conducting observations in a controlled environment. [4 marks]

Controlled environments such as laboratory experiments offer a strong level of control of extraneous variables during observational research. Extraneous variables can interfere or affect the results of the observational research. The removal or minimising of said extraneous variables makes it easier to both establish a causal relationship between the independent and dependent variable and for a later researcher to conduct the same experiment/observation and replicate the same results. This increases both the reliability and the validity of the observational research which could be improved by conducting observations in a controlled environment. (91 words)

11 Discuss research into the influence of early attachment on adult relationships. [8 marks]

Hazan and Shaver (1987) conducted a 'love quiz' in a local newspaper. One section of the quiz assessed the attachment type (secure, insecure resistant or insecure avoidant) between both participants and their parents. The other section assessed their current beliefs about romantic love. The first 620 responses were analysed and researchers found a correlation between people's view of romantic love and their early childhood attachment. Secure children tended to have fully functional, trusting relationships; insecure resistant children were more likely to be extremely worried that they were not loved in their relationships and insecure avoidant children tended to fear intimacy. This provides support for Bowlby's theory that adult relationships are influenced by early attachment/s (internal working models).

However, Freud and Dann (1951) provided evidence that those early attachments may not have as large an effect on adult relationships as Hazan and Shaver's (1987) results implied. They studied 6 children who were orphaned during World War Two and raised in a deportation camp. Although they were cared for by the Jewish people that temporarily lived there, they were unable (due to the short amount of exposure to the adults) to form any adult attachments. However, when the children grew up, they developed average intelligence and were able to form fully functioning relationships. Freud and Dann concluded that this was because they had formed attachments amongst themselves as children. This offers an alternative interpretation of a viable early attachment and its influence on later adult relationships than later attachment styles after a childhood relationship between a parent/adult and a child.

(258 words)

Section D
Psychopathology

*Answer **all** questions in this section*

1 2 Which **two** of the following are examples of Jahoda's criteria for 'ideal mental health'? Shade **two** boxes only. For each answer completely fill in the circle alongside the appropriate answer. [2 marks]

A Dependence on others
B Environmental mastery SHADE THIS BOX
C Lack of inhibition
D Maladaptiveness
E Resistance to stress   SHADE THIS BOX

1 3 Read the item and then answer the question that follows.

The following article appeared in a magazine:

Hoarding disorder – A 'new' mental illness

Most of us are able to throw away the things we don't need on a daily basis. Approximately 1 in 1000 people, however, suffer from hoarding disorder, defined as 'a difficulty parting with items and possessions, which leads to severe anxiety and extreme clutter that affects living or work spaces'.

*Apart from 'deviation from ideal mental health', outline **three** definitions of abnormality. Refer to the article above in your answer. [6 marks]*

One definition of abnormality is a deviation from statistical norms. Behaviour that is rare statistically is considered abnormal within this approach (people on the tail ends of a bell curve graph are statistically rare and therefore abnormal). People with 'hoarding disorder' are '1 in 1000 people', they are statistically rare and therefore abnormal.

Another definition of abnormality is that of an individual being unable to function adequately. Criteria for diagnosis include dysfunctional behaviour (behaviour which contrasts with the cultures accepted and expected behaviour) and personal distress (the individual is excessively emotional, causing themselves unpleasant experiences). In this case, the 'hoarding disorder' is causing the sufferers personal distress i.e. 'severe anxiety'.

Deviation from social norms is a third definition of abnormality. This outlines an individual who contrasts with the expected and accepted behaviours of their society (the social norms). The sufferers of this 'hoarding disorder' are defying social norms as in Western cultures citizens are expected to not have severe problems, 'parting with items and possessions' as the article states 'Most of us are able to throw away the things we don't need on a daily basis'. (186 words)

1 4 *Read the item and then answer the question that follows.*

Kirsty is in her twenties and has had a phobia of balloons since one burst near her face when she was a little girl. Loud noises such as 'banging' and 'popping' cause Kirsty extreme anxiety, and she avoids situations such as birthday parties and weddings, where there might be balloons.

Suggest how the behavioural approach might be used to explain Kirsty's phobia of balloons.
[4 marks]

The behavioural approach may explain Kirsty's phobia of balloons as a product of classical conditioning i.e. Kirsty has learnt to associate balloons with fear. This means that a neutral stimulus (NS) (a balloon) has been presented with an unconditioned stimulus (UCS - loud noise) and produced an unconditioned response (UCR - fear). However, because the neutral stimulus (NS) has been presented and associated with a fear inducing stimulus and response (S+R), the balloon is now associated with the unconditioned (now conditioned) response (UCR-fear). In this way balloons inspire and cause a response of fear in Kirsty. This fear has been maintained through operant conditioning as Kirsty's avoidance of situations where there might be balloons has prevented this conditioned anxiety and fear (CR-fear) from occurring (negative reinforcement) making her more likely to repeat this avoidant behaviour. (135 words)

1 5 Read the item and then answer the questions that follow.

Twenty depressed patients were treated using cognitive behavioural therapy. Over the course of the six-week treatment, each patient's mood was monitored every week using a self-report mood scale (where a score of 20 = extremely positive mood and a score of 0 = extremely negative mood). Each week they also completed a quality of sleep questionnaire which was scored from 10 = excellent sleep to 0 = very poor sleep.

At the end of the study the researchers correlated each patient's final mood score with his or her final sleep score.

1 5-0 2 Outline **one** way in which the researchers should have dealt with ethical issues in this study. [2 marks]

The researchers should have constantly offered or made the participants aware of the right for them to withdraw from the study. This would prevent participant discomfort and distress. (28 words)

1 5-0 3 The sleep questionnaire used by the researchers had not been checked to see whether or not it was a reliable measure of sleep quality.
Explain how this study could be modified by checking the sleep questionnaire for test-retest reliability. [4 marks]

This would be achieved by modifying the sleep questionnaire for test-retest reliability. Firstly, the participants would complete the sleep questionnaire more than once. The scores would then be correlated from each questionnaire. A scatter graph would also be used and on one axis the first tests results and on another axis, the later test's results. This would then be assessed using a Spearman's Rho test and the reliability is then determined by comparing the correlation with the statistical table. It would be expected to display a strong, positive correlation between the two sets of scores. (95 words)

1 6 Outline cognitive behaviour therapy as a treatment for depression. [4 marks]

Cognitive behavioural therapy (CBT) attempts to identify and rectify the patient's faulty cognitions. There are many ways that the therapist and patient can do this. The therapist tries to help the client discern that these cognitions are faulty by questioning them and focussing upon the clients' successes in life. The client may be encouraged to keep a diary to help them become more aware of their thoughts and feelings. The therapy aims to mostly focus on what the client's personal situation is but the therapist may also draw on the client's past experiences. (93 words)

Words: 3377. Copyright: Joseph Campbell 2017.

By Joseph Anthony Campbell

AQA A-LEVEL PSYCHOLOGY (7182/2)
PAPER 2
PSYCHOLOGY IN CONTEXT
SPECIMEN MATERIAL
2017
HTTP://FILESTORE.AQA.ORG.UK/RESOURCES/PSYCHOLOGY/AQA-71822-SQP.PDF

Section A
Approaches in Psychology

Answer **all** questions in this section

0 1 Which **one** of the following statements is **false**? Shade **one** box only. [1 mark]

A Repression can lead to unpleasant memories causing distress
B Repression causes people to have difficulty accessing unpleasant memories
C Repression involves people choosing to forget unpleasant memories   SHADE THIS BOX
D Repression involves unpleasant memories being kept from conscious awareness

0 1-0 2 Which **one** of the following statements is **false**? Shade **one** box only. [1 mark]

A The Id is responsible for pleasure-seeking behaviour
B The Id is responsible for unreasonable behaviour
C The Superego is responsible for bad behaviour   SHADE THIS BOX
D The Superego is responsible for guilty feelings

0 2 Read the item and then answer the question that follows.

In a laboratory study of problem-solving, cognitive psychologists asked participants to solve problems presented in different colours of ink. They found that it took longer to solve problems presented in green ink, than it did to solve problems presented in other colours. They inferred that the mental processing of problems is made more difficult when a problem is presented in green ink.
Explain what is meant by 'inference' in relation to this study. [2 marks]

Inference refers to the assumptions made about mental processes that are not directly supported by evidence. In this context, the psychologists are inferring that because the green ink questions seemingly made the participants solve the problems at a slower rate that they then had more difficulty actually mentally processing the problems.

0 3 Read the item and then answer the question that follows.

Dominic is unhappy and lacks confidence. He also thinks he is not very good-looking and not very clever. He goes to a counselling therapist for help. The therapist suggests that Dominic lacks congruence.
*Outline what is meant by 'congruence'. Explain **one** way in which Dominic might achieve 'congruence'. [4 marks]*

Congruence is the difference between the self as known to the individual and the self the person aspires to become. The therapist could endeavour to bridge the gap between the two incongruent aspects of this self for Dominic by helping him to be able to assess himself more accurately. Through the therapist offering Dominic unconditional positive regard (UPR) Dominic could achieve a more realistic view of himself.

0 4 Discuss the contribution of behaviourist psychologists such as Pavlov and Skinner to our understanding of human behaviour. [16 marks]

Ivan Pavlov carried out an experiment whereby he rang a bell and then provided dogs with food immediately afterwards. The dogs began to associate the bell with food through repetition and soon the bell alone caused salivation. The food was an unconditioned stimulus that produced an unconditioned response (salivation). When the unconditioned stimulus was repeatedly presented with a neutral stimulus (the bell), it was associated with the unconditioned stimulus (the food) and produced a now conditioned response (salivation) and thus became a conditioned stimulus. Pavlov labelled this classical conditioning and it later became known as Pavlovian conditioning.

B.F. Skinner studied how animals and by extension, humans, learn from the consequences of their actions – in particular through positive and negative reinforcement. Positive reinforcement is when something desirable is obtained through the subject partaking in a particular behaviour and Skinner's experiments on rats display this as rats were conditioned to press a lever because it provided them with food, which was desirable. Negative reinforcement describes an undesirable experience or item being removed as a consequence of a particular behaviour and the rats also learnt to press a lever to prevent an electric shock. Skinner labelled this as operant conditioning.

However, although conditioning is supported by evidence, it cannot explain all behaviour. Animals and humans can also learn through observation as demonstrated by the social learning theory. This means that Skinner and Pavlov's theories into conditioning cannot be used on their own to explain all behaviour.

Both Pavlov and Skinner's experiments and much behaviourist evidence relies on animal research. This means that there is a problem of anthropomorphic extrapolation as humans and animals are inherently different in both morals and physicality. Therefore, there is a problem of relating animal studies to humans. Behaviourists seemingly ignore genetic factors also which can impact what different species can learn through conditioning.

Behaviourists also fail to take into account abstract concepts such as morals and also state the 'mind' is irrelevant. Both Skinner and Pavlov fail to outline cognitive processes that take place during conditioning and therefore provide an incomplete explanation of behaviour. It has been applied to classrooms in education and various modes of therapy however and applicability has been found in relation to the real world and it has been useful in understanding certain aspects of human behaviour.

Section B
Biopsychology

Answer **all** questions in this section

0 6 *The electroencephalogram (EEG) and event-related potentials (ERPs) both involve recording the electrical activity of the brain.*
*Outline **one** difference between the EEG and ERPs. [2 marks]*

EEG's show the overall electrical activity in the brain, meaning that it is often used to study sleep patterns.
ERP'S, however, display changes in EEG wave patterns in response to a stimulus, to link certain stimuli to certain responses.

0 7 *Read the item and then answer the question that follows.*

Sam is a police officer. She has just started working the night shift and after a week, she finds that she has difficulty sleeping during the day and is becoming tense and irritable. Sam is also worried that she is less alert during the night shift itself.
Using your knowledge of endogenous pacemakers and exogenous zeitgebers, explain Sam's experiences. [4 marks]

Due to the fact that Sam has been on the night shift for a week her endogenous pacemaker or internal biological clock is out of sync with the exogenous zeitgeber of light. This is because she has to remain awake at night when it is dark and sleep during the day when it is light. This disruption in her sleep-wake cycle has been linked to the problem Sam is experiencing such as difficulty in sleeping and therefore feeling tense and irritable.

0 8 *The human female menstrual cycle is an example of **one** type of biological rhythm; it is called a:*

A circadian rhythm
B infradian rhythm
C ultradian rhythm
[1 mark]

B

0 9 *Outline the structures and processes involved in synaptic transmission. [6 marks]*

When an electrical impulse reaches the end of a neuron, neurotransmitters are released into the synaptic cleft, which diffuse to the postsynaptic membrane. These neurotransmitters might trigger an electric pulse down the postsynaptic membrane therefore continuing through to the synaptic cleft. After the neurotransmitters trigger the electric pulse they are reabsorbed by the presynaptic neuron or broken down by enzymes.

Synaptic transmission occurs at the junction between two neurons. The receptors are on the postsynaptic membranes, which means that the impulses are unidirectional. Excitatory neurotransmitters (e.g. Acetylcholine) make it more likely that an electrical impulse in the postsynaptic neuron will be triggered. Inhibitory neurotransmitters such as gamma amino butyric acid (GABA) make it less likely that an electrical impulse will be triggered in the postsynaptic neuron.

1 0 *Split brain patients show unusual behaviour when tested in experiments. Briefly explain how unusual behaviour in split brain patients could be tested in an experiment. [2 marks]*

Participants who have had split brain surgery could split their visual field by covering one of their eyes in two conditions in a repeated measures experiment and when shown a word or a picture they could report or attempt to draw what they see.

1 1 *Briefly evaluate research using split brain patients to investigate hemispheric lateralisation of function. [4 marks]*

The results found in split brain research cannot always be accurately generalised in order to create nomothetic theories due to their small sample size (for example Sperry used only 11 participants). This means that the findings do not allow for anomalies and therefore they have little practical use. Also, the findings of split-brain patients whom had had drug treatment were compared to an epileptic control group that had not experienced medical (drug) treatment or experienced epilepsy. Therefore, you cannot establish cause and effect between both splitting the brain and impaired function as impaired function may be due to the medication beforehand.

Section C
Research methods

Answer **all** questions in this section

Read the item and then answer the questions that follow.

A psychologist wanted to see if verbal fluency is affected by whether people think they are presenting information to a small group of people or to a large group of people.

The psychologist needed a stratified sample of 20 people. She obtained the sample from a company employing 60 men and 40 women.

The participants were told that they would be placed in a booth where they would read out an article about the life of a famous author to an audience. Participants were also told that the audience would not be present, but would only be able to hear them and would not be able to interact with them.

There were two conditions in the study, **Condition A** *and* **Condition B.**

Condition A: *10 participants were told the audience consisted of 5 listeners.*

Condition B: *the other 10 participants were told the audience consisted of 100 listeners.*

Each participant completed the study individually. The psychologist recorded each presentation and then counted the number of verbal errors made by each participant.

1 2 Identify the dependent variable in this study. [2 marks]

The dependent variable is the verbal fluency of the participants, which could be measured by the number of verbal errors they make.

1 3 Write a suitable hypothesis for this study. [3 marks]

There is no difference in the number of verbal errors made by participants who believe they are reading to a small audience (5 listeners) and by participants who believe they are reading to a large audience (100 listeners).

1 4 Identify **one** extraneous variable that the psychologist should have controlled in the study **and** explain why it should have been controlled. *[3 marks]*

It would be important to control the participant's level of familiarity with the famous author as increased levels of familiarity could decrease the number of verbal errors. This uncontrolled participant variable could affect the dependent variable (DV – verbal error rate) rather than the independent variable.

1 5 Explain **one** advantage of using a stratified sample of participants in this study. *[2 marks]*

Stratified sampling can produce a representative sample of the group you are attempting to generalise the results to. This means that the results may have a higher level of validity when generalising to the general population as different genders male/female are represented in this study sample in the correct proportions.

1 6 Explain how the psychologist would have obtained the male participants for her stratified sample. Show your calculations. *[3 marks]*

60% of the 20 participants should be male therefore 60/100 x 20 = 12
12 participants should be male.
Place the names of 60 males written on a piece of paper in a hat and pick names from the hat until you have withdrawn 12 names. These 12 names are the men that will be used in the sample. Then determine the proportion of males needed to mirror the number of males in the target population as follows i.e. 60%.

1 7 The psychologist wanted to randomly allocate the 20 people in her stratified sample to the two conditions. She needed an equal number of males in each condition and an equal number of females in each condition. Explain how she would have done this. *[4 marks]*

Firstly, the psychologist must write down all the names of the females on slips of paper and put them in a hat. Then the psychologist must randomly withdraw 4 names and put them in condition 1 and then withdraw 4 names and put them in condition 2. The psychologist then must write down all the names of the males on slips of paper and put them in a different hat and withdraw 6 names out of the hat. These will be the participants in condition 1. Then the psychologist must withdraw another 6 names and put them in condition 2.

1 8 Read the item and then answer the questions that follow.

*The results of the study are given in **Table 1.***

Table 1: Mean number of verbal errors and standard deviations for both conditions

	Condition A (believed audience of 5 listeners)	**Condition B (believed audience of 100 listeners)**
Mean	11.1	17.2
Standard deviation	1.30	3.54

What conclusions might the psychologist draw from the data in Table 1? Refer to the means and standard deviations in your answer. [6 marks]

Firstly, the psychologist might conclude that more verbal errors are made when the person believes that they are presenting/reading to a large audience of 100 listeners than if they believe that they are reading to a small audience of 5 listeners. This conclusion is supported by the results of the mean as those in condition A made on average 11.1 verbal errors whereas those in condition B made 17.2 verbal errors on average. The psychologist might also conclude that the differences in participants public speaking skills/anxiety levels became more apparent when participants believed that they were presenting to a larger audience as the standard deviation was larger (3.54) in condition B compared to condition A (1.30).

1 9 Read the item and then answer the question that follows.

*The psychologist had initially intended to use the range as a measure of dispersion in this study but found that one person in **Condition A** had made an exceptionally low number of verbal errors.*

Explain how using the standard deviation rather than the range in this situation, would improve the study. [3 marks]

The range can be easily affected by one anomalous result meaning that the range is easily affected by errors. In contrast, standard deviation measures the average distance of the scores from the mean not just the difference between the highest verbal error score and the lowest verbal error score and is therefore less easily distorted by a single, extreme score.

2 0 Name an appropriate statistical test that could be used to analyse the number of verbal errors in Table 1. Explain why the test you have chosen would be a suitable test in this case. [4 marks]

An unrelated t – test could be used if we record results as interval data (i.e. one verbal error is recorded in the same fashion as another verbal error). The study is also an independent groups design and the psychologist is looking for a difference between the two conditions. All of these factors suggest that the unrelated t-test could be used.

2 1 The psychologist found the results were significant at p<0.05. What is meant by 'the results were significant at p <0.05'? [2 marks]

This means that the researchers would have a 95% confidence level that the results are significant (i.e. the change in the independent variable is the cause of a change in the dependent variable).

*2 2 Briefly explain **one** method the psychologist could use to check the validity of the data she collected in this study. [2 marks]*

They would make the participants take part in a different, established verbal fluency test and check to see the results from both tests are consistent with one another and positively correlated (concurrent validity).

*2 3 Briefly explain **one** reason why it is important for research to undergo a peer review process. [2 marks]*

The peers can check to make sure that not only are the researchers results valid but that the researcher's conclusion/s are supported by their results. This would ensure that the research is less likely to contain any errors when published as it has been independently, objectively scrutinised by peers.

2 4 Read the item and then answer the question that follows.

The psychologist focused on fluency in spoken communication in her study. Other research has investigated sex differences in non-verbal behaviours such as body language and gestures.
Design an observation study to investigate sex differences in non-verbal behaviour of males and females when they are giving a presentation to an audience.
In your answer you should provide details of:
• the task for the participants
• the behavioural categories to be used and how the data will be recorded
• how reliability of the data collection might be established
• ethical issues to be considered. [12 marks]

The participants should give an approximately 10-minute individual presentation to an audience from a script such as 'a list of favourite hobbies' that the psychologists have given them 20 minutes beforehand in order to ensure they have 20 minutes rehearsal time. The psychologists will record the participants' physical language/non-verbal behaviours and then compare the results of the females with the results of the males in order to attempt to find a difference between each gender as regards nonverbal behaviour. The psychologists should record the participants' behaviour using event sampling. Types of non-verbal behaviour must be decided upon and categorised before the study i.e. crossing arms, hand gestures, shifting feet etc.

Each time a participant displays one of these behaviours it would then be recorded on a recording sheet.

The reliability of the data collection could be improved by using two psychologists to record and closely observe the data and then checking the inter-rater reliability between them. Inter-rater reliability determines the levels of concordance between each recorders results and the higher the concordance rate the higher the reliability. A good level of inter-rater reliability is considered to be 80% and anything below this would therefore be considered to have low levels of reliability. Through comparing separate recordings, we can therefore make a statistical comparison of both raters.

Certain ethical considerations must also be taken into account. The participants must be aware of their right to withdraw, have given their informed consent to take part in the study and they must not be entirely deceived as to what the study is researching. These ethical considerations must be in place in order to protect the psychological welfare of the participants and to ensure that they are protected from physical and psychological harm during the study.

Words: 3065. Copyright: Joseph Campbell 2017.

AQA A-LEVEL PSYCHOLOGY (7182/3)
PAPER 3
ISSUES AND OPTIONS IN PSYCHOLOGY
2017

PAPER 3 (A-LEVEL): SPECIMEN QUESTION PAPER (193.6 KB)

Section B
Relationships

0 1 Discuss evolutionary explanations for partner preferences. [16 marks]

Evolutionary explanations for partner preferences are shown through sexual selection. Sexual selection explains certain reproductive behaviours. For example, within a species there are certain characteristics that make individuals attractive to potential mates. This evolution of characteristics which are attractive to potential mates is known as sexual selection. In humans, characteristics affecting attractiveness include physical and mental health and some physical features. These influence potential mates as they indicate an ability to reproduce and provide for offspring.

There are different types of sexual selection. Intrasexual selection which takes place when males compete (often aggressively) and the winner is rewarded with the female. The female is passive in the process and does not choose her own mate. Intersexual selection takes place when males compete for the attention of a female. The female plays an active role, choosing her mate.

Sperm competition is a form of intrasexual selection. Short's (1979) Sperm Competition theory suggests that males are motivated to ensure that their sperm is successful in fertilisation and that they compete against other males to make this happen. In humans this has evolved into men releasing large amounts of sperm during ejaculation. This is a form of intrasexual selection and increases the likelihood of successful fertilisation.

Buss (1989) carried out cross cultural research into intersexual selection. He studied gender differences in mate selection. Questionnaires were used to collect data from over 10000 men and women from 37 different cultural groups. The questionnaires covered demographic information such as age, gender and marital status. They also asked about preferences for variables such as marriage, age difference and characteristics sought in a mate (e.g. intelligence, sociability and financial prospects). The results were that women valued variables associated with gaining resources (e.g. money, safe environment) more highly than men. Men valued variables associated with reproductive capacity (e.g. youth) more highly than women. The conclusion was that women have historically had limited access to the resources needed to provide for themselves and their offspring so they have evolved to select mates who can provide these resources. Men have been limited by access to fertile women and so have evolved to be attracted to women with a high likelihood of reproducing.

Evaluatively the study supports an evolutionary explanation of gender differences in partner preferences. There is high replicability also as similar findings were found across a range of different cultures. However, it was not a truly representative study as it was hard to include rural and less educated populations. The study also did not take social influences on mate selection into account. For example, changes in society mean that women in many cultures are now able to provide for themselves and their offspring and are not as dependent on men for resources. Also, homosexual relationships are not explained as reproduction is not a goal in same-sex relationships.

AQA A-LEVEL PSYCHOLOGY (7182/3)
PAPER 3
ISSUES AND OPTIONS IN PSYCHOLOGY
2017

PAPER 3 (A-LEVEL): SPECIMEN QUESTION PAPER (SECOND SET) (72.7 KB)

Section B
Relationships

Read the item and answer the question that follows.

Teddy is discussing his girlfriend, Sasha. He says, 'We were in the same year at university, both studying marketing. She was really good at the theoretical side and I was better when it came to practical work. We specialise in different areas now. I'm always proud to be seen out with Sasha. Other guys are really jealous when they see her. We tell each other everything though, no secrets in our relationship.'

Discuss factors affecting attraction in romantic relationships. Refer to Teddy's comments in your answer. [16 marks]

It could be argued that we form relationships for selfish reasons. Reward/need satisfaction theory states that we form friendships and relationships to receive rewards or reinforcement from others. Relationships provide rewards (approval, sex, status, love, money, respect, agreement, smiling, and information) that satisfy our social needs for self-esteem, affiliation, dependency and influence for example. Therefore, if we are to apply the model of operant conditioning to this then being in a relationship is positively reinforced because it is rewarding. Byrne and Clore's (1970) Reinforcement-Affect theory suggests that both operant and classical conditioning play a part in relationships. The theory states that we learn to associate people with positive or enjoyable situations even if they are not directly rewarding us in these instances. These associations are powerful in leading us to form relationships with these people.

Filter theory was proposed by Kerckhoff and Davis (1962). It states that we tend to be attracted to those who pass through a series of filters as follows: those who fit a certain social demographic and those we come into contact with who are similar in attitude/backgrounds and those who complement our emotional needs. Filter theory can be viewed in Teddy's comments when he states 'same year at university' which shows similar demographic factors. The Filter theory of similarity is also shown as they were 'both studying marketing'. Finally filter theory's view on complementarity is demonstrated when Teddy states 'She was really good at the theoretical side and I was better when it came to practical work' and that they now 'specialise in different areas'.

Physical attractiveness is also a key component of their relationship as he states that he is 'proud to be seen out with Sasha. Other guys are really jealous when they see her.' The role of attractiveness in relationships links to the matching hypothesis which noted a strong positive correlation between the attractiveness of two partners in a relationship.

Self-disclosure is the sharing of personal information about oneself and increases attraction as shown by Collins and Miller's meta-analysis. Self-disclosure is demonstrated in Teddy's relationship as he states 'we tell each other everything...no secrets'. Self-disclosure is only effective if appropriate to the stage in the relationship – too much self-disclosure too soon has the opposite effect. There is also a difference between the role of factors in initial attraction and their role in continuing this attraction. Kerckhoff and Davis longitudinal study of similarity and meeting needs showed that it was couples who had complementary needs whereby each partner met the needs of the other who were more likely to have progressed towards a permanent partnership.

Reward-need theories also argue that long-term relationships are more likely to be formed if the relationship meets the needs of the two people involved and provides rewards for them. Evidence from Smith and Mackie supports the view that meeting needs, whether these are biological, social, or emotional needs is particularly important in maintaining a relationship.

Words: 1117. Copyright: Joseph Campbell 2016.

AQA A-LEVEL PSYCHOLOGY (7182/3)
PAPER 3
ISSUES AND OPTIONS IN PSYCHOLOGY
2017

PAPER 3 (A-LEVEL): SPECIMEN QUESTION PAPER (193.6 KB)

Section C

Schizophrenia

0 1 Discuss biological explanations for schizophrenia. [16 marks]

Schizophrenia could be caused by biological factors such as genetic factors and inherited tendencies. Gottesman (1991) reviewed approximately 40 twin studies and found that identical twins (MZ; monozygotic) had a 48% concordance rate whilst with non-identical (DZ; dizygotic) twins there was a 17% concordance rate. Evidence for this is presented by Shields (1962) who found that MZ twins raised in different families still displayed a 50% concordance rate. Adoption studies have also found that when children are adopted because one or both of their biological parents has schizophrenia that the chance that they will develop the disorder stays the same despite the change in environment. This suggests a more powerful genetic rather than environmental link to the development of schizophrenia. Gottesman's findings are different however from the Cardno study that found concordance rates of 26% for MZ twins and 0% for DZ twins. One explanation for this difference is that the Cardno study used strict diagnostic criteria to distinguish MZ from DZ twins. Earlier studies did not and so may not reflect the true degree to which genetics explain schizophrenia. The other main issue with genetic explanations is that no single gene has been found for schizophrenia. Studies of mice showing social abnormalities and studies of schizophrenic families found defects in the pp33cc gene; however, this research is in its early stages. Also, no study has found a 100% concordance rate and therefore it is clear that schizophrenia is not simply caused by genes. It may also be a factor that a shared environment may cause higher concordance rates in family studies because children imitate 'schizophrenic' behaviours from their relatives. Therefore, other factors must be considered such as biochemical and psychological factors.

Biochemical factors are supported by post-mortems and PET (Positron emission tomography) scans which have shown that schizophrenics have abnormally high levels of the neurotransmitter dopamine. This has led to the development of the dopamine hypothesis which states that synapses that use dopamine as a neurotransmitter are overactive in the brains of people with schizophrenia. Evidence for this is provided by antipsychotic drugs which reduce the symptoms of schizophrenia by blocking dopamine receptors. This infers that it is the overactive dopamine receptors that are causing the symptoms. Drugs like amphetamines which increase dopamine function can also sometimes cause schizophrenia-like symptoms in people without schizophrenia. However, antipsychotic drugs only work on the positive symptoms of schizophrenia such as hallucinations. This means that increased dopamine function does not explain negative symptoms such as social withdrawal. The link with dopamine is also correlational as it does not show cause and effect. It may be that increased dopamine function is a symptom of schizophrenia rather than a cause of it.

There are neurological factors also such as abnormal brain structure which is caused by abnormal development. Johnstone et al (1976) compared the size of the ventricles in schizophrenics' brains with non-schizophrenics' brains. They deduced that people with schizophrenia had enlarged ventricles which suggests that schizophrenia is linked to a loss of brain tissue. Buchsbaum (1990) carried out MRI (Magnetic resonance imaging) scans on schizophrenic's brains and found abnormalities in the prefrontal cortex. However non-schizophrenics can also have enlarged ventricles which contradicts Johnstone's evidence. These findings are correlational also as they do not show cause and effect; it may be that abnormal brain structure is a symptom of schizophrenia rather than a cause of it.

AQA A-LEVEL PSYCHOLOGY (7182/3)
PAPER 3
ISSUES AND OPTIONS IN PSYCHOLOGY
2017

PAPER 3 (A-LEVEL): SPECIMEN QUESTION PAPER (SECOND SET) (72.7 KB)

Section C
Schizophrenia

0 1 Discuss reliability and/or validity in relation to the diagnosis and classification of schizophrenia. [8 marks]

There are problems with the diagnosis and classification of schizophrenia. Symptoms of schizophrenia may overlap with symptoms of other disorders such as bipolar disorder or symptoms of brain disease or damage. A further difficulty in diagnosis is the stage of the disorder. It is only reliably diagnosed in the active stage where symptoms are numerous and evident. These problems are associated with the classification systems used. In science a good classification system would mean that the categories would be discrete and mutually exclusive but this is not possible with a disorder that has so many subtypes and symptoms.

Reliability is how far the classification system produces the same diagnosis for a particular set of symptoms. In order for a classification system to be reliable the same diagnosis should be made each time it is used. This means that different clinicians should reach the same diagnosis. Validity is whether the classification system is actually measuring what it aims to measure. There are differing types of validity such as descriptive validity i.e. how similar individuals diagnosed with the disorder are, aetiological validity is how similar the cause of the disorder is for each sufferer and predictive validity is how useful the diagnostic categories are for predicting the right treatment.

However, diagnosis might lead to labelling and stigmatisation (Scheff 1966) causing long-term problems of getting/keeping employment and leading to a self-fulfilling prophecy. Rosenhan (1973) conducted a study where people with no mental health problems admitted themselves into a psychiatric unit by stating that they heard voices and thus became pseudo patients. Once admitted they behaved normally but their behaviour was still viewed as a symptom of their disorder by the staff in the unit. This therefore questions the validity and the diagnosis of mental disorders as once people are labelled as having a disorder then all of their behaviour can be viewed through this prism and be interpreted as being caused by the disorder itself. This is a clear example of labelling.

o 2 Discuss token economies as a method used in the management of schizophrenia. [8 marks]

Behaviourists argue that schizophrenia is learnt through operant conditioning. If one receives a positive reaction or reward from others then this encourages the person to repeat the behaviour and it is thus reinforced.

Evidence for this is shown by 'token economies' which use reinforcement to encourage 'normal' behaviour through the awarding of 'tokens' when patients with schizophrenia show desirable behaviour and this can help treat schizophrenia. Evidence suggests token economies can be effective in improving behaviour in psychiatric hospitals. Used for behavioural shaping and management it can ensure that patients in long stay hospitals are easier to manage. Token economics have been used in hospitals and Paul and Lentz (1977) carried out a study to investigate the effectiveness of token economics. A reward in the form of a token that could be exchanged for things they wanted (e.g. cigarettes) was given to schizophrenic patients when they displayed appropriate behaviour such as 'brushing hair'. Paul and Lentz found schizophrenic symptoms did reduce with the use of token economy and this improvement carried on during the hospital stay. This suggests that some schizophrenic behaviour is learnt and is based on Skinnerian operant conditioning principles.

However, patients tended to relapse once out of the hospital and when they were no longer being reinforced for their behaviour. It is also considered these days to be unethical, particularly when trying to shape behaviour using rewards such as food – which is a basic right. Token economies do not address symptoms of schizophrenia also so they are not a 'treatment' and have proven ineffective with unresponsive patients e.g. with negative symptoms. Contrastingly also, the bulk of psychological and biological research suggests that schizophrenia is not just a learnt behaviour.

Words: 1269. Copyright: Joseph Campbell 2016.

By Joseph Anthony Campbell

AQA A-LEVEL PSYCHOLOGY (7182/3)
PAPER 3
ISSUES AND OPTIONS IN PSYCHOLOGY
2017

PAPER 3 (A-LEVEL): SPECIMEN QUESTION PAPER (193.6 KB)

Section B

Gender

0 1 Describe and evaluate Kohlberg's explanation of gender development. [16 marks]

Kohlberg's theory of gender development is cognitive i.e. it involves the brain and its' processes and ways of thinking and relates to the child's understanding of gender. Kohlberg argues that gender development starts at age 2 and finishes at age 7 in the form of three qualitatively different stages. Before a child can progress to the next stage there must be brain maturation i.e. the brain is ready to move on to the next stage.

The first stage is gender labelling and identity (awareness of own gender), which happens between the ages of 2-3 and involves the child labelling their own gender correctly and to recognise other people as male or female. The child bases this on superficial characteristics such as hair length. At this stage the child does not understand that their gender is fixed and believes that they can grow up to be the opposite gender.

The second stage is gender stability and this happens between the ages of 3-6. At this stage the child understands their gender is fixed across time and that, for example, they are male now and will be male when they grow up. However, they may not understand that gender is fixed across situations, for example a man with long hair is potentially viewed as a woman by the child.

The final stage is gender constancy (consistency) and this happens from the age of 7. At this stage the child understands that gender is fixed across time and across situations and they have a more complex understanding of the permanency of gender, understanding that gender is unchanged despite changes in outward appearance (clothing, hair etc.) through understanding gender stability in context. They will also observe models of the same sex to identify gender appropriate behaviours. This is referred to as 'self socialisation' by Kohlberg.

Kohlberg's theory illustrates the processes involved in transition through the stages which involve maturation, socialisation and a lessening egocentrism within the child. His theory of gender attempts to explain the roles of both nature and nurture within gender development also. For example, the process of brain maturation is a biological factor and therefore nature is involved in gender development and nurture is involved in the child's process of self-socialisation. As a result of this, Kohlberg's theory is potentially less reductionist than other theories of gender development such as the gender schema theory. He also has a clear focus on cognition in that thinking governs behaviour which opposes behavioural explanations. Kohlberg's theory is also supported by cross-cultural findings which confirm that the three stages take place in different cultures (Munro et al: 1984).

There is also further evidence to support Kohlberg's proposal that gender development is an active process. For example, Slaby and Frey found that older children with higher levels of gender constancy paid more attention to same-sex models than children with lower levels of gender constancy. This supports Kohlberg's theory that children understand gender differences at different ages and that gender concepts develop through the active structuring of the child's social experiences. This contrasts with the passive learning process proposed by other approaches such as social learning theorists.

Contrastingly, critics argue that Kohlberg has underestimated the age at which gender identity occurs. Research has found that children prefer gender-specific toys at age 2 and children seek out same-sex playmates earlier than the proposed gender identity stage. Kohlberg's theory is also unable to explain why boys show stronger sex-typing than girls. A further criticism of Kohlberg's theory of gender development is that it is considered a good description of how gender develops but it does not offer any real explanation as to how these processes occur. This therefore limits the theory because it lacks depth.

AQA A-LEVEL PSYCHOLOGY (7182/3)
PAPER 3
ISSUES AND OPTIONS IN PSYCHOLOGY
2017

PAPER 3 (A-LEVEL): SPECIMEN QUESTION PAPER (SECOND SET) (72.7 KB)

Section B
Gender

0 2 Read the item and answer the question that follows.

Social psychologists are writing a report about their research into children's toys. They write, 'Parents still tend to buy pink for girls. In fact, it is hard to find any adverts aimed at girls that are not 'pink and fluffy'. For boys, parents tend to buy more competitive or combat-type toys. Good against evil is a common theme in adverts aimed at boys. Even at school, playground activities are different. As children get older, boys and girls tend to have more shared interests like music'.

Discuss the influence of culture and media on the development of gender roles. Refer to the report above in your answer. [16 marks]

Psychological research suggests that culture and media all influence children's development and adoption of gender roles. In terms of cultural influence, in a meta-analysis of 175 studies that analysed how parents treat boys and girls it was found that boys and girls were reinforced differently by their parents for sex appropriate activities. This parental reinforcement is evidenced in the report above as 'Parents still tend to buy pink for girls.' and 'For boys, parents tend to buy more competitive or combat-type toys'. In particular, the meta-analysis found that fathers treated sons and daughters differently than mothers did. Fathers positively reinforced their son's gender appropriate behaviour through their choice of a toy and Segal found that fathers more often responded negatively to feminine play in sons i.e. playing with dolls. These findings support Maccoby who found that parent's reinforced sex typed behaviours, including game and toy choice. Therefore, it could be argued that when gender appropriate behaviour is positively reinforced it will be repeated in the future. Durkin (1995) however, argued that peers are in fact more important in gender role reinforcement than parents. This was supported by Archer who found that children as young as three criticised peers for what they believed to be gender inappropriate play. It appears there is a clear role of direct reinforcement of gender stereotypical behaviours by parents and peers.

Social Learning Theory also argues that reinforcement plays a role and that gender is learned through the observation, identification with and imitation of role models and through witnessing the consequences of gender appropriate behaviour (vicarious learning). There are mediating cognitive variables also i.e. children select which models to imitate by observing parents, siblings, peers of the same sex and/or models who seem to be powerful and/or in control of resources, attractive, similar or of high status for example. Fagot also found more gender role stereotyping in traditional families than in families where parenting was shared. Schools also influence gender roles through teachers as role models, positive and negative reinforcement and as shown in the report schools reinforce different activities i.e. 'Even at school, playground activities are different.'

The media also provides stereotyped gender role models with boy's magazines focusing on sports and computer games, whereas girl's magazines focus on fashion, and relationships. These cultural representations of gender and reinforcement are promoted in various forms of media such as in TV, books and computer games for example. This is evidenced in the report above through stereotypical media representations i.e. the '... adverts aimed at girls ... 'pink and fluffy' and 'good against evil ... adverts aimed at boys'. The inference appears to be that copying the models will result in positive consequences.

Behaviourist and social learning explanations of gender strongly emphasise the role of the influence of society and learning processes and therefore represent the nurture side of the nature versus nurture debate. The implication being that gender roles are determined by social and cultural forces and can change. This is shown in the report above which states that, 'As children get older, boys and girls tend to have more shared interests like music'. This shows that as children grow older; their age can act as a mediating variable which leads to 'shared interests'.

Social constructionists also argue that ideas about gender are constructed and are transmitted through language. There is cross-cultural evidence of differences in gender roles in different societies which supports the view that gender is socially determined. In collectivist cultures the development of feminine traits is encouraged for both men and women, whereas, in individualistic cultures the development of masculine traits is encouraged for both men and women as is evident from Bem's concept of androgyny. Therefore, gender roles vary within, as well as between, cultures.

By Joseph Anthony Campbell

Words: 1424. Copyright: Joseph Campbell 2018.

Printed in Great Britain
by Amazon